RETINAL DETACHMENT

New Information on Retinal Detachment: Causes, Symptoms, and Methods for Patient-Centered Eye Care

CHAD BRUNO

Table of Contents

Introductory

The retina, the light-sensitive layer of tissue at the back of the eye, can become detached from the underlying layers of the eye, causing a dangerous disorder known as retinal detachment. The retina's ability to absorb light and convert it into signals that can be delivered along the optic nerve and into the brain is fundamental to visual perception.

• Small tears or holes in the retina are the most prevalent cause of retinal detachment, while there are other potential triggers. The vitreous, a transparent gel-like material in the eye, can leak through these tears or holes and into the space between the retina and the underlying layers, causing vision loss. If not addressed immediately, this gap might prevent blood and important nutrients from reaching the retina, resulting in vision loss or blindness.

• Flashes of light, a shadow or curtain-like obstruction in the periphery, and the abrupt appearance of floaters (small specks or cobweb-like structures in your field of vision) are all symptoms commonly associated with retinal detachment. If you encounter any of these signs, don't hesitate to contact a doctor right once; timely treatment, usually in the form of surgery, can avoid irreversible damage to your eyes and increase your chances of a full recovery.

The particular therapy for retinal detachment depends on the nature and severity of the detachment but often involves surgery to reattach the retina and heal any tears or holes. It's important to get a full eye exam and start treatment as soon as possible if you suspect you have a retinal detachment or are experiencing symptoms of one.

CHAPTER ONE
Retinal Detachment and Eye Trauma

Retinal detachment, in which the retina becomes detached from the underlying layers of the eye, is a potentially serious eye disorder that may be exacerbated by eye trauma. The retina and other sensitive internal eye tissues are vulnerable to damage from blunt force trauma, such as a blow or injury.

Retinal detachment can be caused by ocular damage in the following ways:

• A tear or hole in the retina can occur if there is sufficient force or stress to the eye. In some cases, the symptoms associated with these tears or holes may not appear until much later. A hole or tear in the retina allows vitreous, a gel-like fluid within the eye, to leak through and collect between the retina and the underlying layers, causing damage to the retina.

• Detachment of the retina can occur if vitreous or other fluids collect between the retina and the underlying layers. Due to a lack of oxygen and nutrients, visual loss can occur if the retina's blood supply is severed.

• Floaters (tiny specks or cobweb-like structures in your field of vision), flashes of light, and a shadow or curtain-like obstruction in your peripheral vision are all symptoms that might result from a retinal detachment caused by trauma. If you've just suffered an eye injury and are experiencing any of these signs, you need to visit a doctor right once.

• Successful repair and preservation or restoration of vision depend on prompt diagnosis and treatment. In many situations, retinal detachment can be repaired with surgery, such as pneumatic retinopexy, scleral buckle, or vitrectomy, depending on the severity and location of the separation.

It is critical to see an ophthalmologist or eye specialist right away if you suffer eye trauma or show signs that could point to retinal detachment after an injury. The chance of irreversible vision loss can be greatly reduced if treatment is administered quickly enough.

Symptoms and Indicators

Retinal detachment symptoms can range from mild to severe and might appear unexpectedly. As retinal detachment is a serious eye disorder that can result in vision loss or blindness if unchecked, it is vital to seek immediate medical assistance if you experience any of the following symptoms. Indicators of a retinal detachment include:

1. Floaters are small, dark spots or specks that appear to "float" in your range of vision and might appear suddenly. Any considerable increase in the size and intensity of preexisting floaters, or the rapid development of many new ones, should be taken seriously.

2. Flashes of Light: Seeing flashes of light, especially in your peripheral vision, can be a symptom of retinal detachment. These glimmers of light could be likened to lightning bolts or brilliant, momentary slashes of illumination.

3. Experiencing a shadow or curtain-like barrier in your field of vision that gradually advances inward is a characteristic symptom of retinal detachment. This visual obstruction may cause some of your eyesight to be compromised.

4. Reduced Central Vision: As the separation advances, you may suffer a loss in central vision, making it harder to see minute details and objects clearly. This can cause a rapid decline in eye sight in certain people.

5. Vision Alterations you may have vision alterations, such as distorted or wavery vision. Objects and straight lines could appear skewed.

It must be emphasized that these signs may also be suggestive of other eye problems. If any of these symptoms appear suddenly, however, you should see an ophthalmologist or other eye doctor very once. Retinal detachment can be successfully treated and eyesight preserved or restored if detected and treated quickly, usually through surgical treatments. Timely care is crucial for optimal outcomes in cases of retinal detachment, which are classified as medical emergencies.

CHAPTER TWO
Evaluation and Diagnosis

A thorough eye examination by an eye doctor or ophthalmologist is often required for the diagnosis and evaluation of retinal detachment. The normal diagnostic procedure consists of the following:

1. First, the doctor will ask you a series of questions about your health, focusing especially on your eyes. They may also inquire as to the presence of any symptoms, such as floaters, flashes of light, or shifts in your field of vision.

2. You will have your central vision tested using a visual acuity chart to see how well you see details up close. This is typically done with the aid of an eye chart, which measures how clearly you can see at various distances.

3. The eye doctor will check the back of your eye, known as the retina, and may do the following tests:

• **Pupillary Dilation:** Your pupils may be dilated using specific eye drops to allow a better view of the retina.

• **Slit-lamp examination:** a microscope equipped with a light source used to examine the anterior and posterior segments of the eye.

Retinal detachments are most common in the retina's outer layers, hence doctors typically employ indirect ophthalmoscopy to investigate these areas.

4. Fundus photography is a technique used to take clear pictures of the retina under certain circumstances. These pictures will be useful in recording the situation and monitoring any changes.

5. Non-invasively capturing high-resolution cross-sectional images of the retina, optical coherence tomography (OCT) scans are a popular diagnostic tool. It can help doctors determine the best course of treatment after determining the severity of retinal detachment.

6. B-scan ultrasonography is a type of ultrasonography used to obtain an image of the eye's internal anatomy by using sound waves. It is especially helpful in situations when cataracts or vitreous hemorrhage make direct retinal viewing difficult.

7. To diagnose your illness, the doctor will ask you about any symptoms you've been experiencing, such as floaters, flashes of light, or a shadow in your periphery.

The results of these tests will help the eye doctor diagnose a retinal detachment, evaluate its severity and pinpoint its location, and decide on the best course of therapy. When identified, retinal detachment is an emergency that requires immediate surgical intervention to reconnect the retina and prevent additional visual loss or blindness. Depending on the kind of the detachment, where it is located, and the patient's overall eye health, a particular surgical method may be used.

Choices in Medical Care

Surgery to reattach the retina and prevent additional visual loss is the standard treatment for retinal detachment. The severity and location of the detachment, the eye's overall health, and the surgeon's skill all play a role in determining the best course of treatment. Retinal detachment typically responds well to the following treatments:

1. Pneumatic retinopexy is a minimally invasive method used to treat retinal detachments that are not difficult and are located in the superior retina. The vitreous cavity of the eye is punctured and a gas bubble is injected there. The patient's head is then placed in a position that facilitates the gas bubble's reattachment of the detached retina. Cryopexy or laser photocoagulation is often utilized to seal the retinal tear or hole. The retina stays linked to the body as the gas bubble is absorbed over time.

2. One surgical option for treating retinal detachment is scleral buckling, in which a silicone band or buckle is put over the affected eye to offer support and reduce the effects of the forces that led to the detachment. As the buckle presses into the eye socket, it releases pressure on the retina. Retinal tears or holes are usually sealed using this method in conjunction with cryopexy or laser photocoagulation. Scleral buckling is typically reserved for retinal detachments produced by tears or holes in the retina.

3. A vitrectomy is an operation in which the vitreous gel in the eye is surgically removed. More serious cases of retinal detachment, such as those complicated by bleeding or proliferative vitreoretinopathy (PVR), a disorder in which scar tissue grows on the retina, may require its usage. Retinal tears can be sealed or the retina can be tamponaded back into place using gas or silicone oil during vitrectomy, giving the surgeon direct access to the retina for healing.

4. Treatment for retinal detachment may require a combination of surgeries in some instances. Depending on the nature of the detachment, a vitrectomy may be followed by scleral buckling or pneumatic retinopexy, for instance.

Your eye doctor will provide a recommendation for treatment

depending on your specific condition. Retinal detachment is a medical emergency that requires immediate attention to increase the likelihood of a successful reattachment and the preservation or restoration of eyesight. After surgery, patients often require intensive follow-up in order to track their recovery and handle any issues that may arise.

Remember that retinal detachment is a medical emergency that requires immediate attention to avoid irreversible vision loss. Seek emergency medical assistance from an eye specialist or ophthalmologist if you suffer any symptoms of retinal detachment, including abrupt development of floaters, flashes of light, or abnormalities in your peripheral vision.

CHAPTER THREE
Methods Other Than Surgery

In most cases, surgery is necessary to reattach the detached retina and restore eyesight after a retinal detachment. However, there are times when non-surgical therapy is an option, either as a stopgap or in certain circumstances.

1. An ophthalmologist may opt to observe a detachment with periodic eye exams if it is minor, located on the periphery, and not associated with considerable visual impairment. This method is mainly reserved for retinal tears that are either asymptomatic or have mild symptoms and are not becoming worse. Surgery may not be required right away if the separation does not worsen.

2. When a retinal tear or hole is discovered at an early stage, it may be possible to repair it by laser photocoagulation or cryopexy (freezing). Due to the intervention involved, these methods are not often included in the category of "non-surgical management," but they are less intrusive than some surgical treatments.

It cannot be overstated that the non-surgical options for treating retinal detachment are highly restricted and not suitable for most patients. To repair the detached retina and avoid additional vision loss, surgery, such as pneumatic retinopexy, scleral buckling, or vitrectomy, is the primary and most effective therapeutic option. In order to increase the likelihood of a positive outcome, early diagnosis and surgical intervention are essential.

Seek immediate medical assistance from an eye specialist or ophthalmologist if you suspect you have a retinal detachment or encounter symptoms linked with this disorder, such as floaters, flashes of light, or abnormalities in peripheral vision. After evaluating your health situation, they will advise you on the best course of action to take.

Methods That Work Together

Combination therapy for retinal detachment may be performed in rare circumstances where a single surgical method may not be sufficient to address the specific characteristics of the detachment. These combined procedures, conducted by skilled ophthalmologists, are always individualized to the patient's specific condition. Some frequent combinations used to treat retinal detachment are as follows:

- Together, vitrectomy and scleral buckling are known as a vitrectomy with scleral buckling. To gain access to the retina without first removing the vitreous gel, a vitrectomy is performed, and then a silicone band or buckle is placed on the exterior of the eye. This method is frequently employed in cases of severe retinal detachment or substantial scar tissue (proliferative vitreoretinopathy).

- Minimally invasive pneumatic retinopexy using laser or cryotherapy involves injecting a gas bubble into the vitreous cavity to reattach the retina. Retinal tears or holes can be sealed with this method, sometimes in conjunction with laser photocoagulation or cryopexy. This combination can be useful for certain forms of retinal detachments.

• Combining a vitrectomy with a tamponade made of gas or silicone oil can help secure the retina in place as it recovers after surgery. Retinal reattachment can be aided by the tamponade's ability to maintain pressure on the retina. Natural absorption of gas takes place over time, while silicone oil is often surgically removed afterwards.

- When several or difficult retinal tears are involved in the detachment, vitrectomy with endolaser photocoagulation or cryotherapy may be necessary. These methods are utilized in the sealing of retinal tears to stop the spread of fluid into the subretinal area.

Each case of retinal detachment is unique, and the surgeon must determine which treatment options will provide the patient the best chance of reattaching the retina and regaining vision. The purpose of combined therapies is to treat retinal detachment from all angles at once.

The particular strategy may vary from case to case, but it is crucial to remember that these combination therapies are normally administered by skilled retinal specialists or ophthalmic surgeons. When retinal detachment is detected, the chances of recovering and retaining vision can be greatly increased with early detection and prompt management.

CHAPTER FOUR
Problems and Results

When ignored, retinal detachment can cause serious consequences and perhaps irreversible visual loss in the affected eye. Treatment outcomes for retinal tears rely on a number of variables, such as the severity of the tear, its position in the retina, how quickly it is detected, and the eye's general health. Retinal detachment can cause the following consequences and effects.

Complications:

1. Scar tissue on the retina and its surrounding tissues can lead to a condition called proliferative vitreoretinopathy (PVR), a serious consequence. Repeated episodes of retinal detachment may result from the scar tissue contracting and pulling on the retina.

2. Macular Involvement: If the macula, which is responsible for central vision and fine detail, is compromised by the detachment, it might lead to irreversible central vision loss or distortion.

3. Retinal detachment can become chronic or recurring, needing several procedures to reconnect the retina, in rare situations.

4. Risks of Surgery: Infection, cataract development, increased intraocular pressure (glaucoma), and lens damage are all possibilities with surgical treatments to reattach the retina.

Outcomes:

- The likelihood of visual recovery is affected by many variables, including as the severity of the detachment, how long it went untreated, how well the surgery went, and how well the eye is doing in general. Early detection and treatment of retinal detachment increases the likelihood of successful visual rehabilitation.

- In other circumstances, the primary goal of treatment may not be dramatic improvement but rather stabilization of the current degree of vision. With stabilization, visual loss can be halted in its tracks.

- Some people may develop lasting visual restrictions, such as impaired peripheral vision, distortion, or decreased contrast sensitivity, even after a successful surgical reattachment.

- It is possible for retinal detachment to return, even if therapy was first effective. Detachments that occur repeatedly could lead to additional procedures and a worse prognosis.

• Surgical dangers Even if the success rates of current retinal surgery techniques have increased, there are still dangers involved in the treatments. One such typical long-term consequence is the formation of cataracts.

It cannot be overstated how vital it is to detect and treat retinal detachment as soon as possible to increase the likelihood of a positive outcome and reduce the risk of complications. When treated quickly, reattachment of the retina and preservation or restoration of vision are often possible outcomes. If you encounter any symptoms of retinal detachment, such as floaters, flashes of light, or changes in peripheral vision, it is crucial to get prompt medical assistance from an eye specialist or ophthalmologist to improve the prognosis and minimize problems.

Protecting Against Retinal Tears and Tear Detachment

Although certain occurrences of retinal detachment cannot be prevented, the risk can be minimized by taking specific precautions and being aware of potential risk factors. Here are some precautions you can take:

• Get your eyes checked regularly by an ophthalmologist or other trained eye doctor. Retinal detachment risk factors and underlying eye disorders can be detected at an early stage by routine eye examinations.

• Follow your eye doctor's instructions for controlling and monitoring preexisting disorders such myopia (nearsightedness), lattice degeneration, and a history of retinal detachment in one eye.

- Wear protective eyewear when engaging in sports, employment, or hobbies that could cause harm to the eyes, such as when dealing with flying debris, sharp objects, or potential trauma to the eye. Eye injuries are preventable with the use of safety glasses or goggles.

- You can reduce your chance of retinal disorders like detachment by keeping your blood sugar levels under control if you have diabetes.

- **Avoid Eye Trauma:** Be vigilant and take safety steps to avoid direct trauma to the eye. You should always take precautions to protect yourself from harm, whether you're in a car, playing a contact sport, or doing anything else that could cause you to sustain an eye injury.

• Having your blood pressure checked regularly is recommended because hypertension is a known risk factor for retinal detachment. Maintaining control of hypertension requires regular monitoring of blood pressure and adherence to advice from your healthcare professional.

• Seek Immediate Medical Attention if You Experience Any Sudden Changes in Your Vision, Such As the Appearance of Floaters, Flashes of Light, or a Shadow in the Periphery of Your Vision. Retinal detachments can be treated successfully if caught early enough.

- **Quitting Smoking:** Smoking increases your risk of developing several different types of eye disease, including retinal issues. The chance of developing these diseases can be lowered by giving up smoking.

- If you wear contact lenses, it is important to take extra precautions to prevent eye infections and complications that could lead to retinal detachment.

- If there is a history of retinal detachment in your family or if you have any other major risk factors, it is important to discuss these with your eye doctor. They can advise on the best ways to keep tabs and stay ahead of potential problems.

Note that while these measures can lessen the likelihood of retinal detachment, they cannot provide complete protection. Retinal detachment can occur in some circumstances for which no known cause can be found. If you suspect you have a retinal detachment, it's important to get your eyes checked regularly and pay attention to any visual problems very away.

Conclusion

The retina is the light-sensitive tissue at the back of the eye, and retinal detachment is a dangerous eye disorder in which the retina gets detached from its usual position. Without quick treatment, this separation might cause permanent vision impairment or perhaps blindness. Visual disturbances such as floaters, flashes of light, and a shadow or curtain-like barrier in the field of vision are common manifestations of this illness.

- Successful reattachment of the retina and preservation or restorations of eyesight depend on prompt diagnosis and treatment. Pneumatic retinopexy, scleral buckling, vitrectomy, and individualized treatment combinations are among surgical methods for treating retinal detachment. Non-surgical treatments are uncommon and reserved for unusual circumstances.

- Treatment results for retinal detachment might vary based on factors such as the degree of the separation, its location, how quickly it is treated, and the eye's general health. Complications such as proliferative vitreoretinopathy (PVR) and macular involvement can occur, and visual outcomes may range from dramatic improvement to stabilized vision or permanent restrictions.

Reducing the risk of retinal detachment entails frequent eye exams, managing underlying eye diseases, safeguarding your eyes from harm, controlling disorders like diabetes and high blood pressure, and seeking fast treatment for any rapid changes in vision.

Warning signs of retinal detachment should prompt a visit to an ophthalmologist or other eye doctor for diagnosis and treatment. In order to treat retinal detachment and increase the likelihood of a positive outcome, early detection and intervention are crucial.

THE END

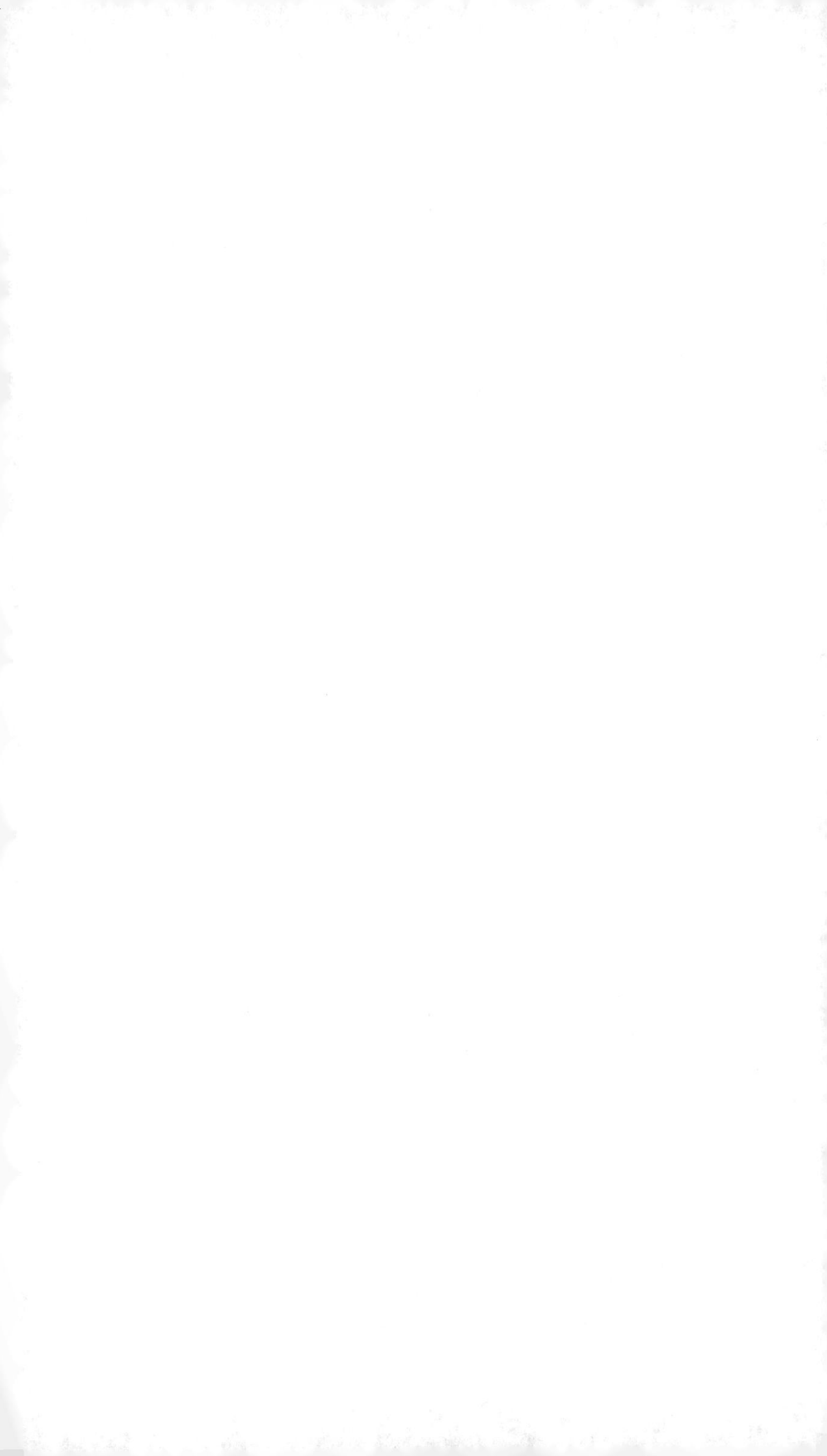